I0420052

Meal Prep

The Essential Guide for Food Preparation and Healthy Eating

Copyright © 2015 by Bora Gyeong

All rights reserved. No part of this publication may be reproduced, distributed, or transmitted in any form or by any means, including photocopying, recording, or other electronic or mechanical methods, without the prior written permission of the publisher, except in the case of brief quotations embodied in critical reviews and certain other noncommercial uses permitted by copyright law.

Disclaimer

This book is designed to provide information on meal prepping. This information is provided and sold with the knowledge that the publisher and author do not offer any legal or other professional advice. In the case of a need for any such expertise consult with the appropriate professional. This book does not contain all information available on the subject. This book has not been created to be specific to any individual's or organizations' situation or needs. Every effort has been made to make this book as accurate as possible. However, there may be typographical and or content errors. Therefore, this book should serve only as a general guide and not as the ultimate source of subject information. This book contains information that might be dated and is intended only to educate and entertain. The author and publisher shall have no liability or responsibility to any person or entity regarding any loss or damage incurred, or alleged to have been incurred, directly or indirectly, by the information contained in this book. You hereby agree to be bound by this disclaimer or you may return this book within the guarantee time period for a full refund.

Table of Contents

Introduction

Meal prepping, also popularly known as "meal prep," is the current trend, and everyone is fighting to get on board, especially those interested in health and fitness. Having caught the attention of many people, its popularity is rising due to the many benefits it has to offer—if the steps are carried out correctly, that is. This should not be taken to mean that only athletes or fitness gurus could benefit from meal prepping, because it is for *everyone*. You might even be practicing meal prepping without knowing it.

It traditionally involves purchasing food in bulk before cooking any of it, then packing into various storage containers. These containers can then be stored inside the refrigerator, and you only need to reheat the portions you want as your meal before eating it. You can prepare a head for a few days.

I am sure you are familiar with the saying, "Failing to plan is planning to fail." Well, this is very true, and it even applies to meals. Meal preparation is important, especially since we live busy lives where we don't have much time to do things that require a significant amount of time, like cooking a meal. Let's say you are working late with a deadline or you are called for an abrupt meeting that ties you up until late—but you haven't done any meal preparation. What will you do if you are single? Maybe you will grab some fast food on your way home. This can end up becoming a behavioral trend. What if you have a family? Then you may decide to whip up something very quick when you get home—anything that takes the shortest time to prepare, such as pasta. Before you know it, you will be feeding your family lots of unhealthy food. Instead of going over all these hurdles, why not get on board with the idea of meal preparation? It is effective, healthy and makes your life much easier.

Meal preparation can work for you, whether you are a working mom, a stay-at-home mom or a full-time student. Don't worry if you haven't tried it out, because we are going to tackle the ways in which you can go about it and the tips and tricks you can use to make sure it works for you.

Chapter One: Benefits of Meal Preparation

How long does it take you to make your meals on a daily basis? This is an important question, because the durations differ for the people who do meal preparation and for those who don't.

The *American Journal of Preventive Medicine* carried an article about a study conducted on the topic of meal preparation. The study involved asking 1,319 adults about the duration they spent in preparing meals, cooking them and cleaning up afterwards. Sixteen percent of the respondents said it took them less than an hour to prepare the food, 43% said they spent between one to two hours preparing food, while 41% said that they spent a minimum of two hours a day on food prep. Where did the difference come from? Some people make earlier preparations and so it takes them a shorter time to do the final preparation before cooking compared to others.

Most people think that you indulge in fast food if you tell them that you take less than an hour to prepare your food. Normally, the people who work from home are the ones who do a lot of meal prepping. However, you can also do it provided you know how to go about it.

Meal prepping and a healthy diet go hand in hand. Therefore, you should spare about half an hour on a weekly basis to do some planning to ensure your family enjoys healthy meals. You may be asking yourself why you should consider meal prepping. These are some of the benefits you stand to gain.

Saves Money

Sometimes, money becomes tight, no matter what you do. It is good to know that you can use meal prepping to save some money, which you can reassign to other equally or more important aspects. This will be possible, because meal prepping enables you to do careful budgeting of your money and planning your meals.

Promotes Healthy Eating

Everyone would like to eat healthy meals, but not all succeed in doing that. For some, it is simply not possible due to lack of prepping. In order to enjoy that meal filled with nutrients, you need to plan. When you get involved in meal planning, you are able to decide on what you'll eat before you even step into the grocery store. Therefore, you get the chance to choose healthy meals for you and your family, as opposed to when you are pressed for time and you end up picking the easiest option or the first food you come across, which may not be healthy. The fact that you can do meal prepping for an entire week means that you can feed your family healthy meals throughout. Normally, when you don't plan for your meals, you end up buying food that you will not eat, and this is a waste of time, money and energy, which you can avoid through meal prepping. This is especially important if you are making a switch to a healthier diet, because planning will help you buy the foods you are supposed to eat and keep you away from temptation.

Prevents You from Wasting Food

We normally waste food when we don't plan ahead. How many times have you discovered a container of food inside your refrigerator that has been there for ages and doesn't look like something that should be eaten? This is what happens when you buy food randomly and some of it gets lost inside the fridge. Meal pepping can help you avoid this, because you will be planning meals for the whole week. Therefore, you will buy what you have planned and you will be forced to prepare them on the particular day of the week you have decided. This means that you will use up all of the food meant for that particular week before buying more. With meal prepping, you can even include a plan for any leftovers, to ensure you don't waste food.

Less Stress

Studies show that stress is very dangerous, especially for your health, so you should always find ways of avoiding it. One way of doing away with stress is by engaging in meal prepping. Imagine it's already evening and then it hits you that your children will soon need to eat something, but you have nothing prepared for dinner? Maybe you are at work, and it seems like you will be getting off late. You have no clue regarding what you and your family will have for dinner and how you'll be able to pull it off. Now that's stressful! If the question that is always on your mind is "What will I cook," then you have some major changes you need to make in your life. This isn't something you should be worrying about on a daily basis. These are some of the circumstances you can avoid when carrying out meal prepping.

A written plan always makes it easier to accomplish anything in any aspect of life and the same applies to cooking. You will be less stressed because you will already know what you are going to prepare in addition to the fact you would be able to do it in a shorter period. It is not even necessary to start the process from scratch on a weekly basis; set a routine that allows you to cook specific foods certain days of the week, and you can regulate the amount of food you use.

Saves Time

This is one of the reasons many people love prepping, especially working moms and busy students. If you have a limited amount of time, especially during the week, then you should find a way to save up some of that time through meal prepping. Imagine the amount of hours you would have spent cooking everything separately for the entire week. When you decide to purchase items in bulk and cook meals one by one, then you save time, because they would only need a very short duration to prepare.

Enables You to Enjoy Variety

If you thought meal planning was rigid, then you should think again. How many times have you found yourself eating the same food over and over again? You may even have French fries for lunch the entire week if you are not keen. However, when you plan for your meals then you are able to accommodate variety. In addition to that, you can add some spices to a simple meal and make it quite different and tastier. For example, you may have prepared chicken squash stir-fry but want it to taste better. You can do this by adding cumin and chili powder to give it a Mexican flavor or you can give it an Indian flavor by adding curry. If you want to make it Italian, then simply add oregano, garlic and thyme. You will find yourself enjoying a variety of food that you will love.

Chapter Two: How to Achieve Meal Prepping

We have already established the fact that meal prepping is very important, and we have examined the benefits you stand to gain from it. The next thing you would normally be thinking of is, "How do I meal prep?" Let's get straight to it.

Invest in Meal Prepping Materials

Before you start meal pepping, you need to have containers that you will be using to store the prepared food. I am not just referring to any containers, but good quality containers. The best examples are the Tupperware or other ones made of glass. It is important to go for containers that are BPA free if you will be reheating the food that is inside the containers. You don't want your containers falling apart inside the oven or microwave. People have different ideas of prepping, and if you are going to do it for some days in a row such as an entire a week, then it is advisable to go for containers of the same sizes. This will make it easy to stack them inside your fridge.

Planning

Meal prepping thrives on planning and so there is no way you can avoid this. Planning is actually the first step towards prepping, so when you have your containers ready, you can begin. If you are a beginner, then you shouldn't overwhelm yourself by cooking meals for the entire week. This is a lot to ask; instead, you can slowly ease into it, because even experts at prepping find it challenging at times. Focus on prepping meals for a duration that you feel is manageable for you, such as a doing it for a few days until you get the hang of it.

Meal planning will help you avoid going to the grocery store and randomly picking up items, then realizing that you won't use them or that most of them are unhealthy meals. When planning, it is important to know the meals you want to prepare and when you would like to do that. Let's say you are organizing meals for about three to four days. You can think of what you would like to serve for breakfast, lunch and dinner. In addition to that, you should also include the type of snacks you will have. After writing down the meals you will prepare, you can then break down the list to include the ingredients you will use to prepare these meals and the appropriate amounts. It is a good idea to start with recipes that you have tried out before in order to avoid buying a bunch of food that you won't find tasty or that you wouldn't know how to prepare. On top of that, try to choose recipes that you can prepare in advance, because that is the whole concept of prepping. Avoid buying foodstuffs that will spoil after a few days. An example of a good breakfast recipe is oats, since they can last a few days in your fridge without going bad.

Prepping

When you have done the necessary preparation, you can actually get down to prepping the food. There are a variety of techniques you can use to prep your food. The main thing is that you should adopt a style that suits your lifestyle, because meal prepping can turn out to be hectic. If you don't do that, then you might give up on it altogether. The first thing you should do when prepping is consider the taste of the food. Everyone loves to eat foods that are both amazing and healthy. Therefore, you should try infusing variety to your foods to make them tastier. For example, you can add some spice coating or sauce to your lean proteins or maybe incorporate olive oil and lemon dressing in your vegetables. This will make meal prepping interesting, because you won't be eating the same food day in day out. Although it is advisable to infuse variety in your diet, it is not compulsory. Therefore, if you are a very clean eater, then you can just stick to what you like best. Having variety should not be a lot of work. Sometimes, it just requires changing some of your protein or spices.

Time

The amount of time you can dedicate to prepping is up to you. This is mostly determined by the amount of time you have on your hands and the amount of prepping you want to do. For example, an individual can prep meals lasting a few days while another can prep meals lasting a week. Therefore, they require different amounts of time. The type of foods you have on your menu will also contribute towards the amount of time you will spend on meal prepping.

You can therefore do it for a whole day or a few hours of the night. Most people find it convenient to prep their meals during the weekends, since that is the time they are free.

If you are prepping meals and snacks that you prefer eating fresh, then you can pack them in the same container and store them in the fridge. It will just be as simple as chopping them up when you want to eat them. Examples of these include salads and veggies. In case you are prepping more complex dishes, then you can chop up the veggies in advance to save you time when cooking the meal. Stir-frys normally fall under this category of complex dishes. Different plans work for different individuals, so it is important to find out what works for you and write it down. It will then be easy to follow that clear plan.

Cooking

All the steps mentioned previously lead to cooking. Meal prepping is meant to give you an easier time when it comes to cooking. This should not be taken to mean that you are supposed to pre-cook everything. You can just do part of the work. For instance, you can marinate chicken breasts before putting them in the freezer. Therefore, you will just need to defrost them whenever you want to use them. You can follow this same procedure for homemade turkey, and so on. Another way method of prepping is to make a bigger batch of sauces that you can refrigerate as opposed to making several smaller batches. For example, you can apply it for your homemade tzatziki, which can be used as a snack when eating your chicken or fish. You can divide your vegetables in different containers, which you would then steam or cook if you prefer freshly cooked vegetables.

If the meal you will be preparing needs a lot of chopping, then do this prior to cooking time. If you plan to have fruits and nuts for snacks, then wash them and have them ready. Some foods can be cooked in advance. Mostly these are good carbohydrates, and examples include brown rice, whole meal pasta and quinoa, among others. This will save you a lot of time, because they normally require long durations of time to prepare.

Chapter Three: Recipes for Meal Prepping

Various delicious recipes can turn the process of meal prepping into a fun one. It is a good idea to experiment with food in order to avoid eating the same thing week after week, regardless of how delicious it may be. You have the ability to transform standard ingredients such as beans, potatoes, and eggs, among others, into something special. These recipes are easy, and you can try them out at home or even get inspired by them to come up with new ones.

Meatloaf Muffins Prepared with Steamed Brown Rice and Served with Avocado

This is a very easy meal to make and is something you can easily take when on the move. In addition to that, you can choose to make a bunch of them and then eat them for days to follow.

Ingredients

- ½ cup of oats

- 1 lb. of ground beef

- 2 tablespoons of oregano

- 1 beaten egg

- 1 cup of organic ketchup

- ½ onion, chopped

- 2 tablespoons of Worcestershire sauce

- Salt and pepper to taste

Directions

1. Heat the oven to 350°

2. Mix all the ingredients inside a bowl, with the exception of ketchup. Make sure they mix well.

3. Divide the mixture and put some into the muffin tin slots.

4. Let the muffins bake for about 20 minutes or until you notice that the beef has turned brown. Take a teaspoon of the organic ketchup and use it to top each muffin.

5. Put the muffins back into the oven and leave them for another ten minutes. Remove them from the oven and let them cool for about ten minutes.

6. Your muffins are now ready and you can pack about 2 to 3 of them for every meal. You can add brown rice and an avocado (half is enough).

Stuffed Sweet Potatoes Prepared with Grilled Chicken Breast

This recipe provides you with variety and is highly nutritious. It consists of foods with lean protein, and the sweet potato boasts nutritional vegetables. Therefore, everyone can enjoy this meal. You can choose to prepare chicken the traditional way or use some tempeh or Portobello mushrooms to come up with something delicious and different. This meal is rich in complex carbs and protein.

This recipe can serve 5 people. It contains 48 g of protein, 2 g of fat and 50 g of carbs, which is equivalent to 405 calories.

Ingredients

- 1 cup of broccoli

- 1 cup of corn

- Chicken breasts, 2 lb. (they should be measured while raw)

- 3 green onions

- Bell pepper, 2/3 cup

- Large sweet potatoes (3 pieces)

- 1 zucchini

- Black beans, 1 cup (this is optional)

- Mozzarella, 5 tablespoons (this is optional)

- Vine tomatoes (2 pieces)

- Various seasonings to taste, such as sea salt, southwest chipotle, cayenne, pepper and paprika

Directions

1. Preheat the oven up to 405°F

2. Wrap the sweet potatoes in aluminum foil. Let them bake until they become soft yet firm, which should be about 45-50 minutes

3. Use the seasonings to season the chicken before putting it into a nonstick skillet to cook. Once cooked, set aside.

4. Chop the vegetables to form small pieces.

5. Take a nonstick skillet and use it to sauté the garlic and corn. Sear before adding in the vegetables and black beans.

6. Slice the sweet potatoes into two before carving out the inside part. Take out the carved out portions and set aside for later use.

7. Spray the sliced sweet potatoes skins with coconut oil before putting them inside the oven for about 5 minutes.

8. Put the vegetable mixture inside the sweet potatoes, and then add about a tablespoon of mozzarella.

9. Let them bake for an additional eight minutes, making sure the oven is at 405°F.

10. Your chicken breasts are ready for serving or you can store some of the stuffed sweet potatoes for later.

One of the reasons people prep food is to avoid waste. Therefore, you can mash up the leftover sweet potato and eat it after adding a couple of ingredients, such as natural sweetener (3 packets), Greek yogurt (1/3 cup), raw honey (1 tablespoon) and cinnamon (1 tablespoon). It tastes good while hot and cold, so you can take it however you want it. If you want to take it for breakfast, then you can heat it up and add some fresh blueberries and granola.

Breakfast Omelet Roll-Ups

You can make your own omelet roll-ups better than the burritos you buy, and they are loaded with eggs rich in protein. They can be eaten as a sandwich, too. This is a very healthy and tasty breakfast.

This recipe is especially great for bodybuilders or those on strict diets where they have to adhere to exact portions. This recipe produces three servings. It contains 1 g of carbs, 50 g of protein, and 11 g of fat, which is equivalent to 350 calories.

Ingredients

- Lean ground turkey, 3 oz

- Goat cheese, 1 oz

- A whole egg

- Bell pepper, 1/3 cup

- 4 egg whites

- 1 handful spinach

Directions

1. Start by seasoning the turkey before coking it in the skillet. Drain.

2. Cook the egg and egg whites in a different skillet.

3. Add the spinach, ground turkey, goat cheese and bell peppers.

4. Roll the mixture before using a plastic wrap to wrap it up

5. Put it inside the refrigerator and just heat it up whenever you want to eat it.

It is advisable to prep only about three of these breakfast omelet roll-ups at a time to ensure they remain as fresh as possible.

Balsamic Chicken

Most of the time, we eat dry, flavorless chicken breasts because we are playing it safe. When you are too safe then, you end up eating an inconsistent diet, which is something you ought to avoid. When preparing your chicken-based meal prep, you can choose to spice it up. This doesn't require much, because the necessary ingredients are probably right in your kitchen. This recipe can produce up to 12 servings. It contains 3 g of carbs, 26 g of proteins and 2 g of fat, which is equivalent to 132 calories.

Ingredients

- Red chili sauce, 1 tablespoon

- Chicken breasts cut to form small pieces, 3 lb.

- Ginger, 1 tablespoon

- Oil-free balsamic dressing, 4 tablespoons

- Honey, 1 tablespoon

Directions

1. Preheat the oven up to 405°F

2. Mix the sauce, balsamic dressing, honey, ginger and red chili inside a small bowl

3. Place the chicken inside a Ziploc bag before adding the balsamic mixture to it. Let it marinate for 20 minutes or more.

4. Put the pieces of chicken on a baking sheet before letting them bake for approximately 12 minutes.

Lean Turkey Lasagna

This meal is perfect, especially if you intend to stay lean while you enjoy the end of the summer. It will make you full while giving you a great beach body, at the same time. It contains 16 g of carbs, 12 g of fat and 55 g of protein, which is equivalent to 387 calories. This meal can make three servings.

Ingredients

- 1 egg white

- Extra lean ground turkey, 1 lb

- Low-fat cottage cheese, 1 cup

- Reduced-fat mozzarella, 1 cup

- 1 zucchini

- Low-sodium basil marinara sauce, 1.5 cups

- Seasonings for meat, such as cumin, garlic powder or onion powder (you may not need seasonings if you buy "seasoned" marinara sauce).

Directions

1. Preheat the oven up to 350°F

2. Use the seasonings to season the ground turkey before cooking it inside a nonstick skillet. The marinara will help to give the meat its sauce so you can add it at this point and then stir.

3. Slice zucchini to form small pieces

4. In a separate bowl, mix the egg white and cottage cheese together.

5. Layer the zucchini inside a small foil tin or jar, adding the cottage cheese (1-2 tablespoons), and then the meat sauce. Do this one more time in order to fill up the jar.

6. Put in one more layer of meat sauce and then, finally, ¼ cup of mozzarella. Do the same for the other two containers.

7. Let it bake for about 30 minutes.

Chapter Four: Tips for Meal Prepping

You may be busy with many things in your life, such as work, family and friends. You cannot be able to eat healthy when you have a limited amount of time. After all, it is easier to order takeout than start thinking about what you will prepare, geting into the fridge or rushing to the grocery store to get food before you can even start the cooking process. Therefore, what would make you resolve to eat healthy meals? The answer is in meal prepping. When you do that, the rest will be easy. Although meal prepping is an interesting task, it can be overwhelming if you don't know what to do. Therefore, you need to have a few tips and tricks up your sleeve that you can use to make the process easier and more effective.

Go to the Grocery Store

The fact that meal prepping will make your work easier doesn't mean you won't have to go to the grocery store. How else would you get your foodstuffs? In addition, don't even talk about online grocery shopping right now. When you are into prepping, you will come up with a shopping list, which will guide you when shopping for foodstuffs at the grocery store. You can choose to get staples because you can work with them to come up with various meals. Examples of what you can get from the grocery store includes tempeh, nuts, bananas, baked chicken, greens, hard boiled eggs, salmon, apples, oatmeal, white fish, protein powder, and so on. This will help you come up with meals such as chicken power a bowl where you simply mix your ready ingredients and cook them using olive oil. Generally, your shopping list will depend on the kind of meals you like and prepare, but the bottom line is that you need to go to the grocery store.

Have Functional Containers

You need functional containers to prep your meals successfully; it is as simple as that. When your containers are empty, you will even feel motivated to fill them up with food. Therefore, this will help you to continue with meal prepping. You should buy containers that can be easily stacked inside your microwave and fridge. They should also be dishwasher friendly and BPA–free. This will save you some space, and it will be easy to clean up. It is advisable to look for containers that best serve your purpose, because different people like to prep different things. You may need to prep some salad that you can take for your lunch, in which case you should consider a container to hold the salad.

Chop Prior to Cooking

If the meal you are planning on preparing requires some chopping, then you need to do this step prior to cooking. This will be your form of prepping. You may not be able to prep the whole meal, and that is why you should prep the basic components instead and store them in preparation for making new meals during the week. If you will be preparing stir-frys, then you need to chop all the vegetables you will be using and have them ready for use. Simply store them in a single container. You can also slice the meat and store it in a different container. When you do this, the main ingredients should be placed into your skillet; cook them for a shorter duration.

Have Your Standbys

You don't need to go overboard when it comes to prepping. Don't start preparing crazy, complicated meals that will come out as a disaster or that you would not be able to eat. You can look for easy and healthy recipes that you can even prepare more than once. This doesn't mean you play it safe all the time, because you need a variety of spicy meals. However, it just means that you should not make the process complicated. For example, you can prepare oats in the evening and grab them in the morning, when you have limited time.

Experiment with Recipes

When you keep flavors simple, then you are able to alter them for the entire week. For example, you can prepare plain chili one night and tacos the next night. You can even add some millet or spaghetti. You can always add new flavors or leave out some in order to come up with something different, almost every time. This will prevent boredom that is normally associated with eating the same meal over and over again.

Start Small

Just like with everything else, meal prep becomes easier with practice. This is why you shouldn't even think of prepping meals for the entire week, because it can be overwhelming. Start small, and you will become an expert with time. For instance, you can begin by learning how to prep eggs, veggies and some snacks. After that, you can move on to some chicken, rice or quinoa and various kinds of foods that you can prep and use during the week. With time, you will know the amount of time you need to prep a variety of things, and you can keep on adding more things, provided you make time. Alternatively, you can do away with some things and only prep what is important to you. Eventually, you will be an expert, and you'll start prepping for the entire week.

Buy a Spiralizer

Sometimes the thought of dicing and chopping vegetables can make the task of meal prepping appear discouraging.

However, you can change this by getting yourself a spiralizer, which will help you prep vegetables in a matter of seconds. In addition to that, it is actually fun to do it. You have a variety of spiralizers to choose from, and you can buy one and incorporate it into your meal prepping. When you do this, you will be increasing your chances of eating healthy meals, because preparing will be easy. This is convenient when you don't have a lot of time to prep vegetables.

Become Familiar with Vegetables

Although spiralizing vegetables is a good idea, not every vegetable is suitable for this. In addition to that, not every vegetable can be kept in the fridge for an entire week before going bad. Vegetables with lots of water go bad quickly, even if you put them in the fridge. If you prep zucchini and cucumber noodles, then do not expect them to last an entire week. However, they can last until the following day. In order to do this, you need to store the sauce separately to avoid it becoming watered down. Most of the vegetables are great for prepped meals, whether raw or cooked. Carrots and jicama are some of the veggies that work well with raw dishes. Parsnips, potatoes and broccoli stems do well with cooked dishes. If you want to come up with collard green wraps, then any type of veggie noodle can do or use your favorite ingredients in preparing sandwiches. Use tinfoil to pack your collard green wraps before storing them in the fridge. They will last an entire week.

This goes to show how important it is to make yourself familiar with various vegetables for correct prepping. When you do this, you will even find it is enjoyable to prepare various vegetables since you will know the proper way of going about it.

Have a Strategy

Having a strategy in everything increases your chances of succeeding, and the same applies to meal prepping. Therefore, you can do this by coming up with a grocery list based on what you plan on having for breakfast, lunch, dinner and snacks too. It is also important to plan for the days you will be eating out, because you will still do that even if you are meal prepping. Having a strategy that caters for food is important, because hunger may strike due to one reason or another, but you will have nothing to worry about if you have food that can last you some days as you sort yourself out. When you have these strategies, you will always go out armed with your snack and so on, which can reduce the temptation to dig in to unhealthy food. If you want to have a successful week, then do not forget about meal prepping—It's a step in the right direction.

Conclusion

Meal prepping can be what you need in your life, especially if you haven't been eating healthy meals. If you always find yourself rushing to the nearest fast food joint to get your lunch or supper, then your deliverance has come in the form of meal prepping. This is something that everyone can do. In addition to that, you have this guide and so you can't go wrong, because it will guide you step by step on how to carry out meal prepping, even if you are a beginner.

Let's say you have a busy morning and fail to get time to prepare a healthy lunch that you can take to work. What will be the alternative? The answer may be to eat an unhealthy meal, which can be detrimental to your health in the long run. Apart from that, we are always looking for ways to save time and money, which are among the most important resources we have—meal prepping can help you do that. When you examine all the benefits associated with it, you do not have an excuse to miss out on meal prepping.

As important as it is to prep food, it is equally important to do it the right way and to consider sanitation. Anything related to food is usually sensitive, and you do not want a scenario where you or your family members suffer from food poisoning. If you are the one handling food, then take the necessary precautions during meal prepping to ensure the food's safety.

It takes time for one to become an expert at food prepping; therefore, do not be hard on yourself when things don't go according to plan. Be patient, and you will soon learn the ropes. For that reason, start small and don't put a lot of pressure on yourself. Everything will work out fine.

Meal prepping is a culture to which you can introduce your family. Therefore, they can even help you out, which will ease your burden, since you won't be doing everything alone. Who says it has to be boring? You can make this a fun and exciting activity that you and your family can enjoy on your way to a healthy lifestyle. Have a great time meal prepping!

www.ingramcontent.com/pod-product-compliance
Lightning Source LLC
Chambersburg PA
CBHW061944280526
45787CB00004B/1717